Best fruits and vegetables to juice for weight loss

By

Joshua A.I.

Table of Contents

Introduction

Fruits and vegetables are packed with essential nutrients such as vitamins, minerals, fiber, and antioxidants, making them an excellent choice for juicing. These nutrients help to boost metabolism, increase satiety, and support overall digestive health, all of which are essential for weight loss. Jump-start weight loss, increase your energy level, clear your mind and increase your overall health as you lose ten to fifteen pounds in just ten days.

"whenever you eat fat, your liver releases bile to break it down and deliver the fat to your body as an energy"

CHAPTER 1:

WHY VITAMINS AND MINERALS ARE THE ANSWER

So Numerous of us wish we had further energy, better abs, and sharper focus. Likewise, we frequently find ourselves wishing that we had better skin or hair. We wish that we could sleep better at night, and wish that it was a little bit easier to wake up (those last two points are related, by the way!). This has led to the emergence of multitudinous diligence, all erected around helping us to feel, look, and perform better. We spend huge quantities of cash on skincare products, on sleep supplements, and on spa enrollments. We try all kinds of crazy effects, whether that's lying on a bed of gentle harpoons to ameliorate sleep (yes, that's a real thing!), wearing blue- blocking tones all day, or wearing energy healing chargers (which are about as effective as wishing really hard!).   We try these effects because we 're looking for answers, and we 're hopeless. We 're willing to try anything. And we hope, each time, that we 're about to stumble upon the answer and unleash our full eventuality. We hope that one of these effects will give the answer and help us feel great as we know that we really can do. But veritably many of these strategies makes any conspicuous difference.   The problem? We 're overcomplicating matters. And this is largely due to the huge quantum of marketing that gets thrown at us on a diurnal base. In verity, perfecting the way you look and feel is veritably simple it's about the basics!

Consider what is very probably to be your modern life-style and your cutting-edge diet. Raise your hand if any of these factors follow to you:

- You don't manipulate your 5 fruits and veggies a day
- You consume a lot of processed meals and prepared foods
- You go to the health club three instances a week or much less – and aren't mainly

cellular the relaxation of the time

- You don't get ample sleep
- You are in a nation of continual stress due to work, family, and economic pressures
- You spend a lot of your free time on the couch, looking at cartoons
- You spend greater than eight hours a day searching at a pc screen, with a hunched back, staring at a shiny display screen
- You spend barely any time outside
- You drink contaminated faucet water
- You breathe dangerous smog-filled air

This is a as an alternative bleak picture, however it's real for MANY of us. We don't devour sufficient greens, we don't sleep, we gorge on sugary foods, and we're harassed all the time. Then we marvel why we don't sense 100%!

Even if you obtained most of these matters right, the reality is that our present-day existence is simply in reality horrible for our health.

This is really proper down to the truth that most of us are too relaxed – we have end up "adapted" to a comfortable, domesticated lifestyle, and consequently our bodies have forgotten how to deal with stress or difficulty.

Take going outside for instance. Most of us simply don't do this enough, which capability that we aren't getting the necessary stimulus of sunlight, which helps to inspire the physique to produce diet D, which in flip regulates matters like hormone production, sleep, mood… even appetite!

Without that necessary enter (called an "external zeitgebers" in the scientific literature) our physique loses some of its herbal rhythm and sure approaches are interrupted.

But then there's the big gain of being in the cold. Even when the solar isn't out, being outside helps to raise testosterone levels, support our immune system, and even enhance our capability to adjust our personal physique temperature.

Is it any surprise we continually experience "stuffy" when we in no way instruct this phase of our health?

Even spending time barefooted on the earth (which trains tiny muscular tissues in the foot), even diving into water and protecting our breath (which trains our lungs and improves our CO2 balance) … these are all matters our bodies crave. And we aren't giving them that.

And our bodies are deteriorating hugely as a result. Compare a wolf in the wild to an overweight, spoiled home dog. Which is healthier?

You are that home dog. Plus, an extraordinarily worrying life-style and lack of sleep…

STARTING WITH VEGETABLES AND FRUITS IS THE SOLUTION

Starting with veggies and fruits is the solution. Why?

Well, it's all very top and nicely me telling you that you need to be working out all through the day, and that you must be ingesting perfectly, and that you need to be taking long swims in freezing bloodless water in the morning. Problem is, we don't have time for that and our bodies are now so maladapted that they wouldn't manage it.

Even fixing your weight-reduction plan – getting rid of all that undesirable processed food, decreasing the wide variety of whole calories, getting extra fiber, lowering easy carbs… it's a lot of work and can get pretty complicated. Which is why the pleasant location to begin is by using fixing one of the largest troubles with present day life. That is: the lack of micronutrients.

Micronutrients are vitamins, minerals, amino acids, fatty acids, antioxidants, and different lively substances in our meals that our physique makes use of for a extensive range of distinctive purposes.

What many humans don't comprehend is that we actually are what we eat. You hear this a lot; however, many human beings expect that it is a variety of metaphor. But no: your physique takes in the vitamins that you eat and then it makes use of these vitamins to virtually rebuild your body.

For example, your bones are made partly from calcium, and magnesium. These additionally assist to fortify your connective tissue (tendons and ligaments), your teeth, and your nails. Connective tissues in a similar fashion gain from the likes of collagen (found in bone broth) which additionally helps to enhance your skin.

If solely you ought to get extra fruit and greens in your eating regimen then, you would turn out to be the healthiest and most positive model of yourself. And that in flip would possibly then provide you the strength and strength of mind to do the rest.

Fruits and veggies can even supercharge your metabolism, assisting you to burn via plenty greater fat!

As we will see in the relaxation of this book, fixing your consumption of fruits and veggies doesn't want to be difficult. If you are strategic, then making simply a few easy adjustments can seriously change your fitness and wellbeing.

This e book will additionally define many of the different exquisite and complicated methods in which fruits can enhance your fitness and overall performance – some of which are sincerely transformative to the way you seem to be and feel.

You'll comprehend exactly which fruits and veggies you want to treatment any of your present-day maladies, and you'll recognize exactly how to get them.

Let's get to it.

CHAPTER 2:

AN INTRODUCTION TO VITAMINS

Before we go further, let's observe extra carefully the precise advantages of fruits and vegetables. And of course, the first vicinity to begin is via searching at the diet content.

It may additionally shock you to understand that nutritional vitamins have been determined much less than a hundred years ago. Until they had been formally discovered, docs knew that positive meals helped with sure bodily conditions, however they did now not apprehend why.

For example, the British Navy carried a provider of limes as early as 1975 due to the fact docs had located that consuming a positive quantity every day, or consuming the juice, stopped sailors from getting scurvy.

However, it used to be now not till 1912 that Casimir Funk, working in the UK then later in the USA got here up with the time period "vitamins," which later grew to be vitamins. The learn about of nutritional vitamins has improved considering that that time, and whereas most of us be aware of the names of the most frequent vitamins, we might also no longer constantly apprehend what they do. There are two kinds of vitamins. These are fats soluble nutritional vitamins and water-soluble vitamins.

Fat soluble nutritional vitamins are these nutritional vitamins that the physique is in a position to store. This capability that if you do now not use all of the nutritional vitamins that you consume, they can be saved in the physique for use when the physique is in want of them.

The apparent benefit of fats soluble nutritional vitamins is that if you're eating regimen is quickly missing in one of these vitamins, you are much less probable to go through a deficiency. That downside of these sorts of nutritional vitamins is that if you eat too lots of one of them, then your physique is unable to flush out the surplus and you may want to go through from a diet overdose.

Fat Soluble Vitamins

The most frequently acknowledged fats soluble nutritional vitamins are diet A, diet D, diet E and diet K.

Vitamin A helps to preserve the pores and skin moisturized, as properly as making sure that the mucus membranes stay moist, supple and smooth. It additionally helps to keep healthful eyesight in low light, as properly as maintaining the reproductive device wholesome and promotion healthful bone growth. Sources of diet A encompass complete milk, butter, eggs and liver. A structure of diet A, carotenoids are located in red, yellow and darkish inexperienced veggies and fruit.

Vitamin D is vital for the physique to take in calcium. Therefore, it is accountable for wholesome tooth and bones, simply like calcium. However, each are wished and work together. Vitamin D is frequently brought to 'fortified' ingredients such as fats spreads and cereals. It is additionally regarded as the sunshine nutrition as the foremost supply of nutrition D comes from sunlight. Vitamin E is accountable for preserving wholesome muscles, apprehensive device and reproductive system. It is additionally an anti-oxidant. Being fats soluble, it is saved in the physique and can assist to defend physique cells from the results of free radicals, which be detrimental to different physique cells.

Sources of diet E consist of entire grains, nuts, wheat-germ oil and inexperienced leafy vegetables. Overdosing on diet is idea to be dangerous. Vitamin K is usually accountable for blood clotting. Without it, each and every time you reduce yourself you would be in hazard of bleeding to death.

This diet additionally makes kidney tissues and bone. Sources of diet K encompass liver, cheese, cereals, darkish inexperienced leafy greens and fruit. It is additionally made in the intestines by using pleasant bacteria.

Water soluble nutritional vitamins can't be saved in the body. This potential that if you devour too plenty of one of these vitamins, the quantity that is no longer used is excreted thru urine. The benefit of water-soluble vitamins is that you are not likely to go through from an overdose.

The downside of these nutritional vitamins is that you may additionally want to take in large quantities as it can't be stored. If your food regimen is poor in one of these vitamins, even for a quick time, you may additionally go through signs and symptoms of diet deficiency as a result, there is no again up grant saved in your body.

Water Soluble Vitamins

The most usually be aware of water-soluble nutritional vitamins are diet C, and the whole team of B vitamins. Vitamin C is additionally recognized as ascorbic acid. It helps to hold the body's connective tissues, that is, the muscle, fat, and bone framework.

It additionally helps to heal wounds with the aid of rushing up the manufacturing of new cells, is an anti-oxidant, and helps the physique to take in iron. Another characteristic of diet C is to guard the body's immune machine enabling it to combat infection.

Sources of nutrition C consist of fruit, fruit juices and vegetables. The B crew of nutritional vitamins consists of B1 or thiamin, B2 or riboflavin, B3 or niacin, B6 or pyridoxine and B12 or cyanocobalamin. This crew of nutritional vitamins is surely worried with retaining the physique functioning properly.

Vitamin B1 is necessary in supporting the physique to metabolize electricity from fats, alcohol and carbohydrates. Sources of this nutrition are lean pork, unrefined cereals, seeds and nuts.

B2 helps the physique to use and digest carbohydrates and proteins and continues a wholesome appetite. Sources of B2 consist of fish, poultry, meat, milk and eggs. Brewer's yeast is a properly supply of this vitamin, as are darkish leafy vegetables.

B3 is necessary for perfect increase and enabling oxygen to glide thru physique tissues. It is additionally accountable for preserving a healthful appetite. Sources of diet B3 encompass fortified bread and cereals and meat.

B6 is accountable for acquiring vitamins and power from the meals we eat. It helps stop coronary heart disorder through getting rid of extra homocysteine from the blood. Sources of B6 encompass soya beans, means, nuts, eggs, entire grains, fish, lamb, port, rooster and milk.

B12 helps to make wholesome crimson blood cells. It additionally permits the physique to transmit messages between the body's nerve cells, enabling us to hear, move, assume and regular day-to-day activities. It is made by way of microorganism in the body's small intestine.

This nutrition is introduced to many foods, such as cereals, and even though it is a water-soluble vitamin, it can be saved in the liver. Sources of B12 include poultry, fish, milk, meat and eggs. The best way of ensuring that you take in enough water soluble and fat-soluble vitamins is to eat a balanced diet. If you think that you may be deficient in some vitamins, you should consult a doctor for advice.

CHAPTER 3:

AN INTRODUCTION TO MINERALS AND OTHER AMAZING NUTRIENTS IN FRUITS AND VEGETABLES

Whereas fruits are generally packed with vitamins, minerals have a tendency to come more so from our greens – although make no mistake, each fruits AND veggies are packed with both.

So, a right query to begin with may be: what is the distinction between a diet and a mineral?

Whereas nutritional vitamins are natural and thereby are generally pretty risky (they can be damaged down by using the likes of heat, air, and acid), minerals are conversely inorganic. In fact, a mineral can sincerely be a steel or a rock

– something you would by no means surely suppose of as being a critical constructing block in what makes you.
But certainly, minerals are integral to the healthful characteristic of the human body. Iron for instance is a vital mineral that the physique makes use of to make hemoglobin

– the crimson blood cells that tour round the physique carrying oxygen.

Without this process, it would be not possible to supply electricity round the physique for the infinite integral features that go on – which include breathing, digesting, and more.

Typically, minerals have a tendency to have a barely greater essential function in the structural factors of the human physique – and the more difficult elements. For example, minerals structure bones, tendons, and ligaments.

Minerals additionally play a position in conduction, however. The physique is powered by using electrical energy after all, and retaining the right cost is necessary for the healthful feature of our muscle mass and brain.

That's why an improper stability of sodium and potassium can motive cramping, as the physique is unable to ship messages effectively to the muscles. Likewise, a lack of calcium can limit power as it is wanted to manage the cost in the muscle cells.

Did you know? You can inform the distinction between a fruit and vegetable based totally on the seed/stone. Vegetables don't have them! Foods that have shocking categorizations include: tomatoes (fruit), coconut (fruit), avocado (fruit), and cucumber (fruit).

Other Essential Micronutrients

As properly as being prosperous in nutritional vitamins and minerals, fruits and veggies are additionally a wealthy supply of the two different necessary nutrients. The different indispensable vitamins are: vital fatty acids, and imperative amino acids.

The time period "essential" capacity that these materials can't be synthesized within the body, and so consequently need to be received from our diet. And possibly this ought to additionally be a clue as to how large a hassle it is that 99% of us are now not getting them that way!

So, what do these vitamins do?

Well, amino acids are in actuality the constructing blocks of proteins. We get a lot of these from meat, and our our bodies will then smash down these constituent components in order to rebuild our tissue. As we noticed at the begin of this book, we actually are what we eat!

This is why amino acids and proteins by using extension are so necessary for bodybuilders and athletes attempting to construct muscle.

Research suggests that the most useful stability for athletes is 1 gram of protein for each and every 1lb of bodyweight. Protein additionally has different advantages – it is tons tougher to convert into fats for instance, and it has a thermogenic impact that means that in reality digesting it will surely burn calories!

Thus, many humans will be challenging at work making an attempt to locate sources of protein from meat and will consume giant quantities of hen to construct better muscles. This can come to be tough work! But what they forget about is that veggies and even fruits additionally incorporate protein (though greens are barely choicest in this sense).

Don't simply remember the protein you obtained from that protein shake and chicken, assume about how an awful lot is in the broccoli on the facet of the chicken.

Amino acids additionally play a host of different roles in the physique and are used to produce digestive enzymes, neurotransmitters (brain chemicals) and a good deal more. They can additionally do matters such as creating.

Finally, fruits and veggies comprise indispensable fatty acids. These are necessary fat that assist us to higher take in different fruits and vegetables, and additionally serve a vary of extra beneficial advantages – such as improving talent characteristic (the talent is made of a giant quantity of fat!).

Omega three is one of the most effective vital fatty acids there is and has a HUGE host of incredible benefits. Often, we suppose of omega three as being something we get from fish, however in reality it additionally exists in desirable quantities in seaweed, hemp seed, walnuts, kidney beans, soybean and more.

CHAPTER 4:

FRUITS AND VEGETABLES FOR ATHLETIC PERFORMANCE

When you suppose of an eating regimen for constructing muscle, your thought likely turns to the traditional options. Your probable will focal point specially on protein sources like chicken, tuna and eggs. An athlete's eating regimen must consist of nothing however meta and steamed rice, right?

But this is a way from the solely type of meals that's going to be beneficial for constructing muscle and enhancing performance. In fact, for bodybuilding, sprinting, swimming, long-distance running, and any different sort of athletic pursuit it is tremendously vital that you get a balanced food plan that will include a extensive vary of one of a kind meals groups. In particular, it is necessary you get your fruits and vegetables.

Interested in taking dietary supplements to raise your athletic performance? What may pastime you to analyze is that ingesting fruits and veggies can simply be greater high quality whilst additionally costing tons much less and having a myriad of different extraordinary fitness benefits!

Here are some examples.

Top Fruits and Vegetables That Improve Athletic Performance

Beets

Beets are a long way and away amongst the very most essential veggies for constructing muscle and for athletes of all kinds.

That's due to the fact beets are amongst the most high-quality meals in the world when it comes to elevating nitric oxide. Nitric oxide is a herbal 'vasodilator'. This capability that it can reason the blood vessels (veins and arteries) to dilate (widen) thereby encouraging the glide of oxygen and vitamins round the body.

The end result is that the muscle tissues get greater oxygen and power at some point of coaching and greater vitamins for improving recovery. This can assist you carry for extra reps, run similarly distances and get better at a quicker rate.

Potatoes

Carbohydrates are frequently made out to be the terrible guys however in truth they are very vital for constructing muscle and for bodily coaching in general. Potatoes are a true preference of carbohydrate due to the fact they're additionally excessive in fiber, excessive in diet C (which enhances recovery) and low in calories. Consume after a exercise and the electricity will go straight to the muscular tissues instead than the waist.

Spinach

Spinach is a vegetable that is excessive in protein as properly as being an accurate supply of phytoecdysteroids. These don't have something in frequent with anabolic steroids however they may additionally have a comparable impact

– with some research suggesting they are an excellent choice for encouraging muscle constructing and testosterone production.

Kale

Kale is the vegetable absolute best in calcium. Calcium is definitely very necessary for your workouts; no longer solely does it assist to enhance the bones however it additionally reinforces your connective tissue and it helps to toughen contractions for greater explosive electricity at some point of workouts.

Kale is very ultra-modern proper now being excessive in protein and low in calories. A disgrace it fees a truthful bit though!

Mushrooms

Mushrooms are technically no longer fruits or vegetables, however they are located in the equal aisle and they're secure for vegans, so they're honest recreation to consist of here. Mushrooms are now not solely any other tremendous supply of protein however additionally come with a vast vary of extra fitness advantages and advantages. They're packed with minerals; they can motivate healing from education and a lot greater besides!

It's without a doubt solely a count of time till we begin seeing mushroom protein shakes cropping up in fitness stores!

The different outstanding gain of mushrooms is that they include nutrition D. In fact, they're one of the few dietary sources of diet D! (Another being oily fish).
This is vital seeing as nutrition D is regarded to be a grasp hormone regulator, and is accountable for encouraging the manufacturing of testosterone in specific – one of the predominant anabolic hormones for constructing muscle and burning fat.

What's more, is that nutrition D has lately been proven to be a good deal greater effective than even diet C when it comes to helping the immune device and stopping colds and flus. As any athlete knows, a bloodless can be ample to entire derail and athlete's education plan, which in flip can be the distinction between victory and failure!

Carrots

Carrots are commonly healthful and a wonderful supply of diet A, C and K. What's genuinely interesting about them even though is the lutein, which can also assist to expand power ranges and beautify the effectivity of your very mitochondria!

Your mitochondria are the electricity factories of your cells which convert glucose into ATP (glucose being the sugar that comes from carbs, and ATP being the usable structure of electricity in your body). This in brief capability that with carrots and different sources of lutein, you can simply run quicker and that you'll in reality burn greater energy even when you're resting!

In one study, rats had been given lutein (which wishes a supply of fats to soak up such as milk) and it was once located that they started out going for walks lengthy distances voluntarily in their wheel, burning a lot of greater fats as they did.

Apples

Apples are wealthy in diet C, which is any other indispensable nutrition for bettering the immune device and supporting athletes instruct longer and more difficult besides fail. Vitamin C additionally helps to motivate the restore of muscle tissue, will increase serotonin to resource with intellectual recovery, and even will increase the manufacturing of each testosterone and nitric oxide when paired with zinc.
On pinnacle of all this, apples are also very wealthy in fiber, which can assist to enhance bowel movements, the absorption of food, blood pressure, and more. Fiber is additionally key to aiding a healthful microbiome, which in

flip can aid a wholesome immune system, higher mood, weight loss, and a good deal more.

CHAPTER 5:

AMAZING SUPERFOOD FRUITS AND VEGETABLES FOR MOOD, ENERGY, BEAUTY, AND MORE

So, you're now not specifically involved in weight loss? Perhaps you are already pleased with the measurement you are? (Good for you!)

Maybe you're no longer an athlete? Maybe you don't have major fitness problems?

Look, fruits and veggies are for everyone. And just to ram that factor home, right here are some greater examples of fruits and veggies with wildly various extraordinary wholesome benefits Broccoli and Leafy Greens for Beauty and Pregnancy
Yes, fruits and greens can assist to make you seem extra beautiful. And that's proper even of something as easy as your humble broccoli!

Broccoli is possibly a little much less 'exotic' when in contrast with some of the different superfood fruits and greens on this list. But don't let that idiot you: this is nonetheless a distinctly nutritious meals that anybody have to be getting greater of.

For starters, broccoli is a properly supply of fiber and can as soon as once more assist to enhance your digestion, your bowel movements, and a great deal more. On pinnacle of that though, broccoli is additionally very excessive in nutritional vitamins K, nutrition C, fiber, potassium, collagen, iron, calcium, and more.

Let's begin by means of diving into that collagen. This is something that all of us want however very few of us get. Collagen has been proven to enhance talent feature and fight towards Alzheimer's, it additionally helps to limit again pain, improves pores and skin elasticity, strengthens the nails, combats leaky intestine syndrome, fights knee pain, and normally toughens up your tendons, ligaments, and bones.

This is why ingredients such as bone broth as so relatively top for us. And now latest lookup is suggesting an even extra effective purpose that collagen would possibly be so important. Researchers now suspect that human beings would as soon as have lived chiefly by using ingesting bone marrow from animal carcasses. The argument goes that hunter-gatherers can also have been ill-equipped to take on massive prey. However, we have been very suitable at monitoring down our prey and following them.

What probable would have befallen often, is that we would have observed antelopes and different animals to the factor the place they had been attacked and killed with the aid of animals like lions and tigers. They would then have stripped these animals of all their meat, leaving in the back of the skeleton. That's when the foxy and imaginative people would have come along, damaged open the bones with our tactile hands, and then eaten the nutritious collagen from inside.

If this is certainly true, then we developed in surroundings the place we bump off massive quantities of the parts of bone. And we now locate ourselves flung into a world the place we very not often get these vital nutrients. If that's the case, then broccoli may additionally be even greater advisable than we at first assumed!

Pregnant moms have to truly appear into consuming greater broccoli and extra vegetables in general. That's due to the fact each broccoli and many salad leaves are a top supply of folate, which is something that all moms are endorsed to eat.

Not getting adequate folate will increase the threat of problems in pregnancy, and that's why a lot of moms will strive and get extra artificially thru the use of being pregnant supplements.

This is the place it's essential to factor out the big blessings of getting extra vitamins from your weight loss program alternatively than from supplements. While it's proper that you can advantage from supplements, the clue right here is in the name. These are supposed to complement your everyday diet.

That is to say that they must be taken in addition to your normal diet, as a substitute than as an alternative. Nutrients from your eating regimen are some distance extra fantastic than these taken in tablet form, as they are mixed with several different nutrients, fats, fibers, and different elements.

Together, these assist to enhance absorption of the key elements and that makes them a whole lot extra effective. The factor to understand is that the human physique developed whilst being uncovered to these ingredients and consequently is optimally designed to extract the dietary price in this form.

It is no longer designed to eat vitamins in a artificial form. This is why so many inform you no longer to take nutrition capsules on an 'empty stomach'. They simply work higher as foods.

Cayenne Pepper for Weight Loss, Testosterone, and More

Cayenne pepper in the meantime is every other tremendous device in the war in opposition to inflammation. This is a compound that makes meals spicy and is broadly located in ointments and lotions due to its anti-inflammation effects. It's a frequent pain relief too as it depletes nerve cells of the chemical 'substance P'. Substance P reasons each infection and the sensation of pain, so this is a super factor to add to your food plan if you do go through from a circumstance like fibromyalgia or arthritis.

Cayenne additionally comes packed with flavonoids and carotenoids. These are antioxidants that stop cell damage, thereby similarly combating towards inflammation.

Cayenne pepper additionally has a range of different outstanding benefits. It has been proven to be an wonderful urge for food suppressant for instance, which means that if you are any person who struggles to stick to a diet, you would possibly begin discovering it a little simpler to be disciplined and thereby optimistically see the weight start to fall off.

At the identical time, cayenne pepper may additionally assist to enhance digestion. This is necessary due to the fact higher digestion doesn't solely supply you extra electricity and stop discomfort, but it additionally helps you to higher take in vitamins from your food. That capacity that all the advantages you're getting from the different superfoods on this listing will then be became up to eleven

What's extra is that cayenne pepper has additionally been proven to extend testosterone. This of direction is the hormone that most of us be aware of as the 'male hormone' and is accountable for the male intercourse drive, as properly as many of the variations between guys and women. Increasing testosterone in guys will increase muscle tone, reduces fats storage, raises aggression, aids with recovery, fortifies the immune device and more.
Men who don't get adequate testosterone will show off symptoms of depression, low energy, low mood, and low intercourse drive. They additionally warfare with weight reap and low muscle mass. Conversely, guys with excessive testosterone showcase the characteristics that we companion with the basic 'alpha male' alongside with toned and effective physiques.

This is why so many guys strive to increase their herbal testosterone manufacturing via the use of steroids and different pills – regardless of these carrying severa fitness warnings and serious dangers.

The simply annoying phase is that testosterone in guys is growing throughout the globe via 1% a year. This is partly due to the use of female merchandise and their influence on our water, alongside with a host of different troubles (certain plastics and our typically inactive lifestyles). But weight loss plan performs a BIG section in it too. Time to begin ingesting a little much less processed food, and a little extra cayenne pepper.

Elderberry for Inflammation

Elderberry is a berry that is wealthy in nutrients. It is as soon as once more a fruit that is absent from many of our everyday diets, and so it's one that you have to think about reintroducing.

The easy truth of the be counted is that most of us remember on the identical few fruits and veggies day in and day out. This way though, we are making sure we get a lot of vitamins in effect, whilst lacking out on some others. The fantastic weight-reduction plan is the most assorted weight loss program – the one that consists of the largest vary of special fruits, vegetables, meats, herbs, and more. So, what can elderberry do for you?

Elderberry has been used in view that prehistoric instances and has been used as a complement or remedy with the aid of a host of historic cultures – inclusive of the Ancient Egyptians. Today we now understand that these fruits are exceedingly excessive in flavonoids and mainly our pal's anthocyanins – effective antioxidants like resveratrol.

At the equal time, elderberries have been proven to assist improve the manufacturing of cytokines. These are the messenger molecules that our bodies use in order to manage the immune system. Pro inflammatory cytokines assist to inspire inflammation, whilst anti-inflammatory cytokines assist to limit them. This is all very necessary due to the fact it essentially ensures that the physique is in a position to accurate alter its personal response to viruses and diseases, and to assist heal wounds and injuries.

Many of us suppose that infection is continually a awful element – in reality though, irritation helps to wreck infections earlier than they have a risk to take effect, as nicely as to inspire recuperation by means of turning in extra vitamins to the affected area. The hassle is when this response goes haywire.

It turns out that for comparable reasons, elderberry would possibly additionally be distinctly nice at combating allergies!

On pinnacle of all this, elderberries are additionally notably superb at combating and destroying pathogens, being beneficial in conflict infections, colds, and a host of different problems. Most fascinating of all, the tiny berries incorporate effective antiviral dealers that have been proven to sincerely 'deactivate' viruses.

These work by way of stopping the viruses from being in a position to damage thru cellphone partitions the usage of their haemagglutinin spikes, which in flip renders them nearly inert. They are accordingly very high-quality for combating troubles like rhinitis, as properly as stopping them from happening in the first place.

Of course, there is additionally the standard nutrition and mineral content material that you have a tendency to get from berries.

CHAPTER 6:

HOW ANTIOXIDANTS HELP YOU TO LIVE LONGER

Antioxidants are discovered naturally in our food regimen and are additionally a key characteristic of many a supplement. Antioxidants are something of a buzz phrase these days and antioxidant nutritional vitamins and minerals as nicely as a vary of Naka Herb dietary supplements are enormously popular.

What is the motive for this? And what exactly are antioxidants? Here we will seem to be a little at how a mobile phone works, how a mobile die and why antioxidants are so important.

Our cells are made up of a number of components however all you want to recognize about in this occasion is the mobile wall and the nucleus. The telephone wall, surrounded with the aid of mitochondria, is the phase of the cellphone that of route holds the entirety collectively and offers the cellphone its spherical appearance.
Meanwhile the nucleus is the core of the cell, which is frequently referred to as the 'control center'. In right here is the place the DNA is stored, the 'blueprint' that tells the phone what it appears like, how to behave and the place the different vital cells go in the body.

Unfortunately, even though what's additionally in our physique is 'free radicals' and this is the place the antioxidant nutritional vitamins and minerals and the Naka Herb dietary supplements come in. Essentially free radicals are supplying that tour round the physique and injury the cells. They are a spinoff of many matters from certainly respiration (oxygen is reactive and damages cells) to getting too lots direct daylight (the UV waves in the daylight are radioactive and can harm our cellphone partitions too).

These free radicals then do a lot of serious injury in the physique and are sufficient to in the end make our pores and skin seem older – due to the fact the injury even though microscopic can sooner or later add up to be seen to the bare eye and this goes for pores and skin cells as well. This is why a lot of publicity to the solar will make you seem excellent and tanned in the quick term, however subsequently end result in your pores and skin performing wrinkled and leathery.

More critically though, ultimately these free radicals will damage all the way via the cellphone walls, and this will imply that they attain the nucleus the place the DNA is housed. If they attain this then they can reason harm to your genuinely genetic code and this effects in mutation which modifications the expression of the phone and renders it unable to do its job.

Because cells reproduce by means of splitting (mitosis) this then capacity that when the mobile splits it will reproduction the DNA throughout and you will have two fault cells. Your immune gadget tries to cease this and can be aided if you purchase herbs online, however it would be higher of direction if it may want to be prevented. Because these lifeless cells as they unfold grow to be cancer, and can in the end lead to the failure of total organs.

Antioxidant nutritional vitamins and minerals from fruits, vegetables, and even dietary supplements will assist you to do this – by way of destroying the free radicals on have an impact on thereby stopping them ever inflicting that damage. These will then sluggish your seen ageing and assist to deter most cancers – no longer bad!

CHAPTER 7:

HOW TO USE FRUITS AND VEGETABLES TO SUCCESSFULLY IMPROVE YOUR HEALTH

At this point, you need to have a complete thinking of the quality motives to make sure you are getting adequate fruits and greens in your diet. These can decorate your fitness in a myriad way, and if you are presently feeling tired, moody, unwell, or even depressed, it's quite probably that you have a deficiency in at least one of these micronutrients. And this need to come as no surprise – given that the sizeable majority of humans DO have some sort of deficiency these days.

The subsequent query is how you must be gently integrating these fruits and vegetables. Are there any drawbacks? How many do you want precisely? Can you simply use a diet pill instead?

How Many Fruits and Vegetables Do You Need Really?

You would possibly have heard that you ought to be aiming to eat at least 5 unique fruits and greens a day. This is a piece of conventional recommendation that is given by using many fitness groups and governments. Some corporations have accelerated this quantity to seven. It is suitable advice, then again it is additionally arbitrary.

What do I suggest by means of that? Essentially, that it is based totally on nothing!

Fruits and greens are now not inherently true for you. They are now not right for you because they are fruits and vegetables. Rather, they are correct for you BECAUSE they incorporate all these fundamental micronutrients.

Those micronutrients are required in unique portions and varieties, and in the end the exceptional issue we can do for our health is simply to get as many of them as possible. The greater fruits and greens you consume, the better. And it is very tough to overdose when you get your vitamins from herbal sources like this.

And be very doubtful when a packet of meals tells you it counts as "one of your 5 a day." If that meals is particularly processed, then probabilities are it won't incorporate many vitamins in it at all anymore. At the very least, it is possibly to be a whole lot decrease in fiber.

Thus, the advantages won't be as notable as they would have been had you ate up that nutrient itself. Apply some frequent sense, and the place possible, devour as many whole, actual fruits and veggies as you can!

The Dangers of Too Many Fruits and Vegetables

That said, you can do yourself harm by using eating too many fruits and vegetables. Or to be a little greater specific, it is notably handy to purpose damage with the aid of eating too lots fruit.

That's due to the fact fruit is rather acidic and packed with sugar. Both these matters make it detrimental to your tooth in particular. Many human beings who change to diets that are notably focused on the use of smoothies will cease up creating serious enamel problems!

One answer to this is to keep away from ingesting too a great deal fruit juice or too many fruit smoothies. Instead, focal point on ingesting vegetable smoothies, which commonly comprise a lot much less sugar.

Another consideration is that fruits and greens are nevertheless a supply of calories. This is specifically real for matters like avocados, which have come to be all the rage recently. While avocados are exceptional for boosting testosterone (thanks to their healthful saturated fats content), and whilst they are beneficial for these attempting to avoid carbs, they can nevertheless make you fat!

Don't make the mistake of questioning that "fruits and greens are healthful and consequently can't make you fat."

The fact is that they nevertheless incorporate energy and you nonetheless want to song and control these energies to keep away from undesirable weight gain.

CHAPTER 8:

CREATING A DIET RICH IN FRUITS AND VEGETABLES

So, you want to be ingesting greater fruits and vegetables, and we've viewed already that there are a big range of unique meals that have a specially incredible advantage – simply as there are a big quantity of particular nutritional vitamins and minerals that you want to attempt and are searching for out in your diet.

But how do you go about imposing that plan? How do you go from struggling to get your 5 a day, to being capable to without problems eat a giant plethora of exceptional really helpful ingredients?

Because that's the different key component to realize: you shouldn't be taking a reductive method of making an attempt to are trying to find out every object individually. If you do this, then you'll locate that you give up spending a massive quantity of money, and finally now not getting a great deal benefit.

This e book has listed a big wide variety of fruits and veggies that you can are looking for out mainly in order to revel in advantages for your beauty, for your power levels, for inflammation, for immunity…You would possibly consequently be tempted to assume you can pick out and pick out the advantages you want! But this is the incorrect approach.

When there are that many distinctive superfoods that every provide some sort of remarkable benefit, you surely can't be trying to find out every one individually. This is specifically genuine seeing as many of them won't combine together, many aren't reachable in your neighborhood supermarket, and some will solely be safe to eat for a brief quantity of time. So, what do you do instead?

The Strategy: The Aim is Variety

Instead of looking for out person one of a kind fruits and vegetables, what is a way preferable is to surely goal to get the largest range you maybe can in your diet. By doing this, you will cowl the biggest spectrum of ingredients, and thereby get the greatest vary of distinctive advantages from your diet.

You ought to locate the healthiest superfood vegetable in the world, however if that was once all you ate then you wouldn't get all that tons gain – due to the fact you'd solely be getting giant quantities of these equal ingredients.

We don't assume of meals such as apples as being wonderful foods, however due to the fact they include giant quantities of diet C (antioxidant, boosts testosterone, encourages nitric oxide formation, produces serotonin), epicatechin, they are simply as brilliant as these extra exclusive ideas.

Moreover, if you consume three extraordinary fruits and vegetables, then the vary of vitamins you get will be a way greater.

Studies exhibit as well, that our microbiome – the healthful microorganism dwelling in our guts – gain most of all from a various diet. The larger the vary of ingredients you eat, the enhanced your intestine fitness will be – ensuing in weight loss, greater energy, higher mood, and more. Finally, by means of aiming to simply "eat plenty of fruits and vegetables" you can limit the quantity of concept this weight loss program raise involves, which in flip will assist you to be extra in all likelihood to stick to your new commitment.

How to Increase the Variety of Fruits & Vegetables

So how do you amplify the variety? Here are some handy pointers that will assist you to do that barring including a lot of stress to your subsequent purchasing trip:

•	Make a lot of stews, hot pots, and Italian dishes. If you're cooking something like a bolognaise, then it's without a doubt very effortless to simply throw a bunch of fruits and greens into a pot with some mince.

•	To make this even easier, strive grating matters like carrot (so you don't want to peel), and use frozen components like mushrooms, peas, and sweetcorn.

•	Make a lot of salads! a convenient way to make a bloodless lunch is to get some salad leaves, throw on some candy potatoes, slice some cucumber, and add a pinch of lemon. This can go on the aspect of almost anything you cook. Choose toddler leaf spinach and you'll get iron and folate. Then simply differ which leaf you use each and every time.

•   Freeze! When doing this, prepare dinner up giant batches of meals and then freeze them in loads of for my part portioned Tupperware's. Then all you want to do is to defrost every one as you come to devour it.

•   Make smoothies! These are extraordinarily convenient to produce – simply throw a bunch of fruits and/or veggies in and hit blend. They additionally furnish a large raise of remarkable benefits. Some of the liveliest and completely happy humans I comprehend eat each day smoothies!

•   Buy fruits and greens out. A lot of cafes promote fruits at the counter, and the equal is proper in many grocers. Instead of shopping for a chocolatey snack, simply purchase the most exotic-looking fruit you can find!

CHAPTER 9:

WHAT ABOUT MULTIVITAMIN SUPPLEMENTS?

If the most important advantages of fruits and veggies come from the vitamins, minerals, and different integral micronutrients, then you would possibly have a very lifelike question: what about multivitamins?

A multivitamin complement is a complement that carries a stability of exceptional nutrients. You may generally see one that carries a mixture of nutrition C, D, A, and B complex. Likewise, multimineral dietary supplements would possibly comprise Iron, Magnesium, Potassium, Calcium, and Zinc for "healthy bones and hormone balance."

Are these merchandises simply as proper as the "real deal?"

Yes and no.

On the one hand, you can soak up and gain from supplements. Some humans will inform you that this isn't true, however there are various appropriate motives to accept as true with otherwise. For one, did you recognize that there really exists numerous merchandise that are designed to change your whole diet? These consist of the likes of Soylent, which supposedly consists of each and every single nutrient the physique needs, all balanced perfectly.

Is it a suitable idea? Not at all! But the aspect to focal point on proper now is that humans who use this product survive… and they're absolutely pretty healthy! And with that in mind, we can consequently country for positive that multivitamins can additionally be absorbed.

But there's a catch. The first of these catches is that a multivitamin is solely going to be as appropriate as the individual who designed it. We noticed with lutein and different fat-soluble nutritional vitamins for example. These want a supply of fats in order to be absorbed into the bloodstream. Get them from herbal meals sources, and possibilities are that the supply of fats will be included. Get them from a nutrition complement and they may not.

Similar interactions additionally exist between many different nutritional vitamins and minerals, the place one will assist the different to be absorbed greater easily. Likewise, one of a kind nutritional vitamins and minerals soak up at distinctive rates, and so ideally shouldn't be blended into a single product.

Then there are all the different matters that fruits and greens incorporate that do us desirable – such as fiber, amino acids, and more. PLUS, there's the small truth that all fruits and veggies include supplies that we don't utterly recognize or possibly aren't even conscious of.

We solely simply found the exquisite advantages of lutein (that go past eye health). So consuming actual fruit and greens is always preferable.

But with that said, if the desire comes down to the usage of a complement or no longer getting those advisable vitamins at all… then the complement is of direction better. In fact, a complement can be a very handy and handy way to get what you want in your diet, or can be regarded as a "back up."

CHAPTER 10:

CONCLUSION - YOUR BLUEPRINT FOR GREATER HEALTH

And with that, we attain the quilt of this guide. At this point, you need to now have a lot higher notion of exactly which fruits and veggies you want in your diet, which ones can grant the most benefits, and how it's without a doubt the range of these matters that trumps the whole lot else.

Likewise, you have to now have a grasp of the pleasant approaches to get these fruits and greens in your diet, and the quality approaches to keep away from any troubles that can come from them.

With all that said, right here is your blueprint to improve your fitness and happiness vastly with the aid of getting extra fruits and vegetables:

- Start your day with a smoothie, however don't have greater than one fruit smoothie

- Don't purpose to get simply 5-7 fruits and veggies in your diet. Get as many as you can in order to get a assorted mix.

- Use a complement as a "back up." This is additionally in particular beneficial when searching for out extra difficult to understand and uncommon nutrients.

- But make certain that you study the directions and do your very own research. You might also desire to assume about timing and including a supply of fats to resource absorption.

- Use techniques to make it as handy as viable to get extra fruits and veggies in your weight-reduction plan

- Avoid processed meals and "empty calories" – exchange matters like chips and chocolate bars with salads and carrot sticks

- Maintain this application for 30 days. You must discover you observe you have greater energy, drive, and higher health.

- Use this new strength to enhance your life-style in different ways!